HAND TOOLS

Images for Reflection & Reminiscence©

First published by Dog Ear Publishing
4010 W. 86th Street, Ste H
Indianapolis, IN 46268
www.dogearpublishing.net

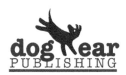

ISBN: 978-159858-731-9

This book is printed on acid-free paper.

Printed in the United States of America

Dedication

Originally, I was going to dedicate this book to my dear parents, Dorothy and Jack Koffman who were married for almost 60 years. Dad was diagnosed with dementia in the 1980s and passed away in the 1990s. Mom was his primary Caregiver for all but the last few months of his life. She passed away just one day short of six months later.

For years, my younger sister Judy was right there on the front lines for the folks . . . my other siblings and I did what we could in support of them.

In the years since my folks' passing, I have focused on community work on behalf of seniors. It has become crystal clear to me that the primary Caregiver has the hardest task and deserves the support and acknowledgement of the entire family.

And so, that is why this book is dedicated to you . . . the Caregiver . . . I know my folks would approve.

To you has fallen the important and difficult – and beautiful – task of being there to assist your Special Senior day in and day out.

It is my sincere hope that this book will give your Special Senior many moments of peaceful reflection and fresh reminiscences.

Please know that these moments are for you as well.

As an addition to the dedication, I want to acknowledge my incredible wife, Sandy. You are my dearest, closest friend, life and business partner, fellow adventurer and dreamer. You illuminate my life with your warmth and compassion. I love you for eternity.

Message to Caregivers and How to Use This Book

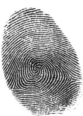

The specific experiences of a person with dementia are as unique and individual as that person's thumbprint.

The forms of dementia are many, varied and ever-changing, but it is still possible to have moments of loving closeness, happiness, sharing and joyful connectedness, no matter the depth of the dementia.

There may be images in this book that will spark reflection and fresh reminiscences in your Special Senior. It is my sincere hope that this will be so.

As your Special Senior looks at the images, watch closely . . . Do they linger or smile while on a particular page? . . . Take that as your cue to ask a simple question: "What does this remind you of?" or "Tell me something about this." . . . Then listen and see what happens . . .

Several pages at the end of the book have been left blank for you to add specific images of other HAND TOOLS that may have personal meaning for your Special Senior. We suggest that these images or photographs be simple and not include people or other details that could be distracting or cause confusion or frustration. We also suggest that only copies of original photos be used and that they be well secured to the page. Again, watch closely for a cue and ask a simple question . . . Then listen and see what happens . . .

The *Simple Pleasures for Special Seniors*© book series has been designed in a straight forward, respectful and friendly manner in order to facilitate special moments of joyous connection between you and your Special Senior.

Enjoy every precious moment of joyous connection . . . and treasure every day!

HAND TOOLS IN THIS BOOK

HAMMER
SAW
SLOT SCREWDRIVER
PHILLIPS SCREWDRIVER
DRILL
CLAMP
PLIERS
LOCKING PLIERS
ADJUSTABLE WRENCH
LEVEL
PRYBAR
WORK GLOVES
LONG NOSE PLIERS
PUTTY KNIFE
TAPE MEASURE
WIRE STRIPPER
RAZOR CUTTER
PENCIL

For more information, Hard Cover Editions or to contact Dan Koffman visit
www.SimplePleasuresforSpecialSeniors.com

Simple Pleasures for Special Seniors©
Titles in Soft Cover Editions now available at
www.amazon.com and www.barnesandnoble.com
FRUITS, FUN FOODS, HAND TOOLS

Simple Pleasures for Special Seniors©
Titles coming soon

**VEGETABLES, DESSERTS, ICE CREAM, COCKTAILS, IN THE KITCHEN,
IN THE GARDEN, SPORTS BALLS, GONE FISHING, FIXING CARS** *and many more . . .*

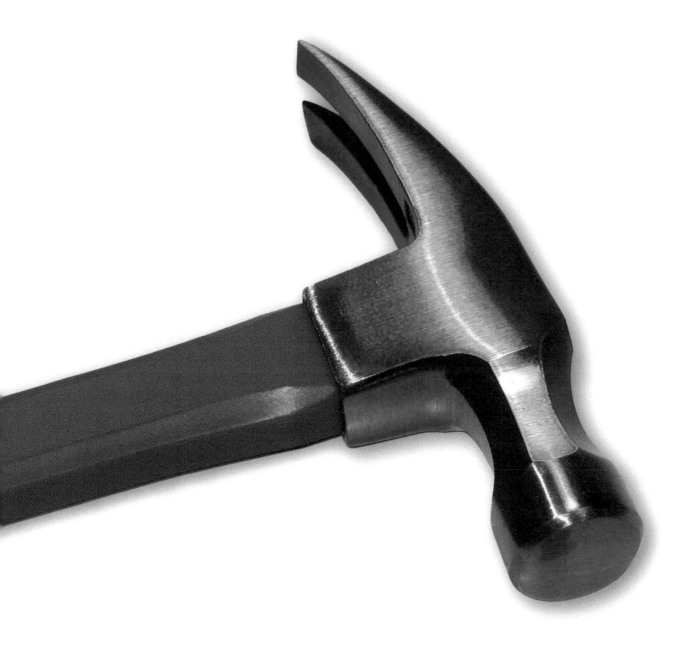

HAMMER

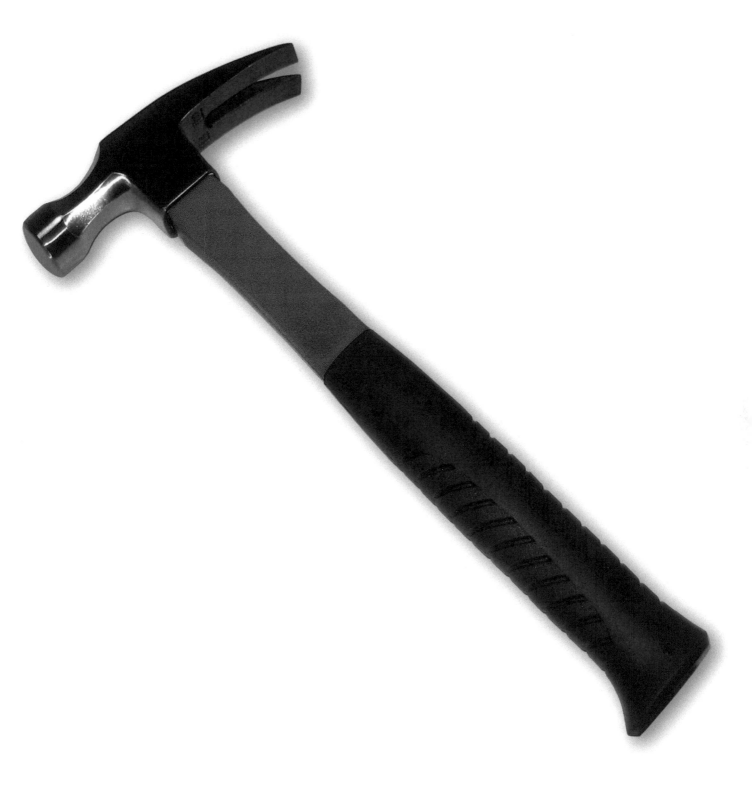

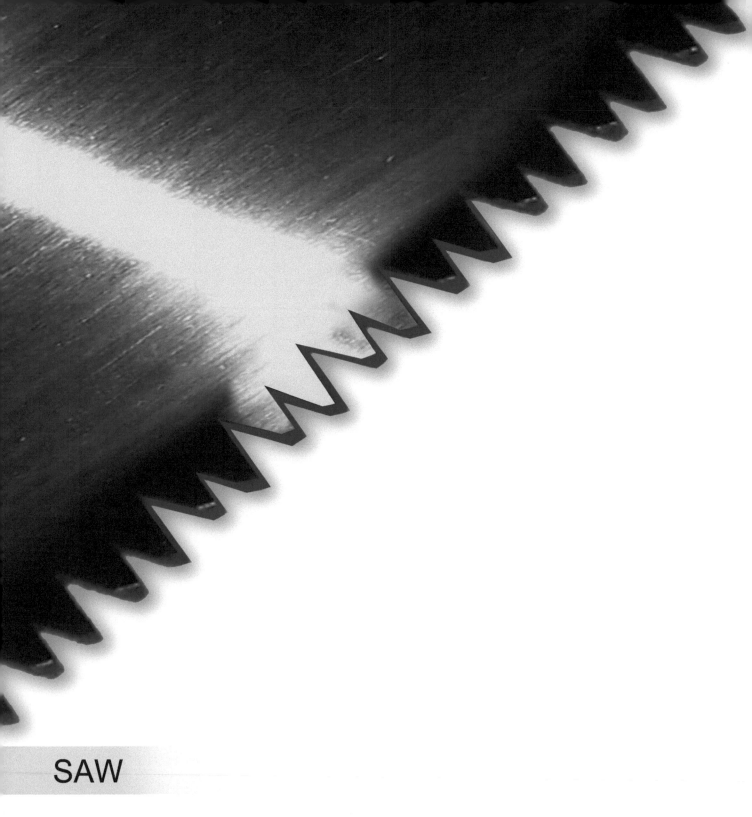

SAW

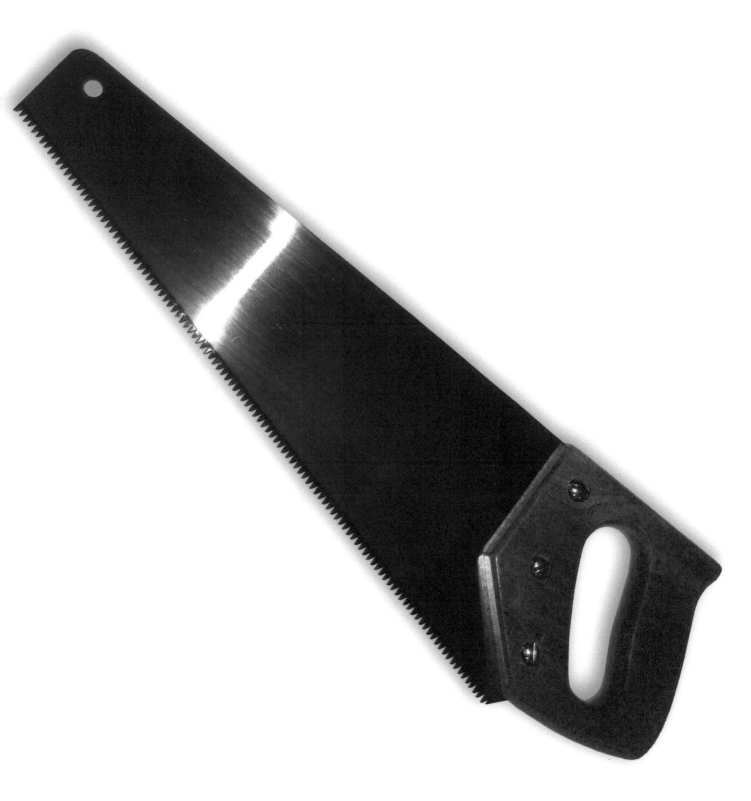

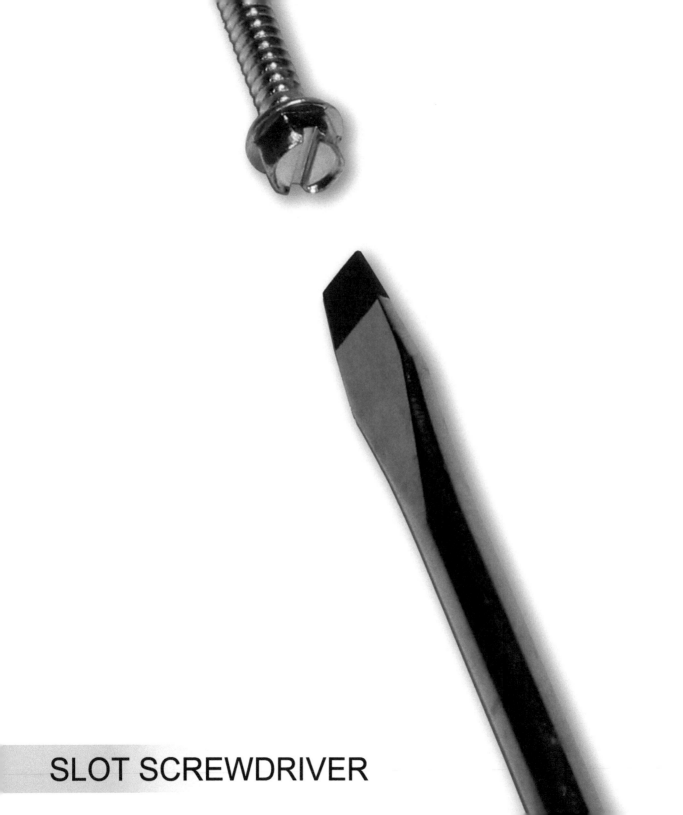

SLOT SCREWDRIVER

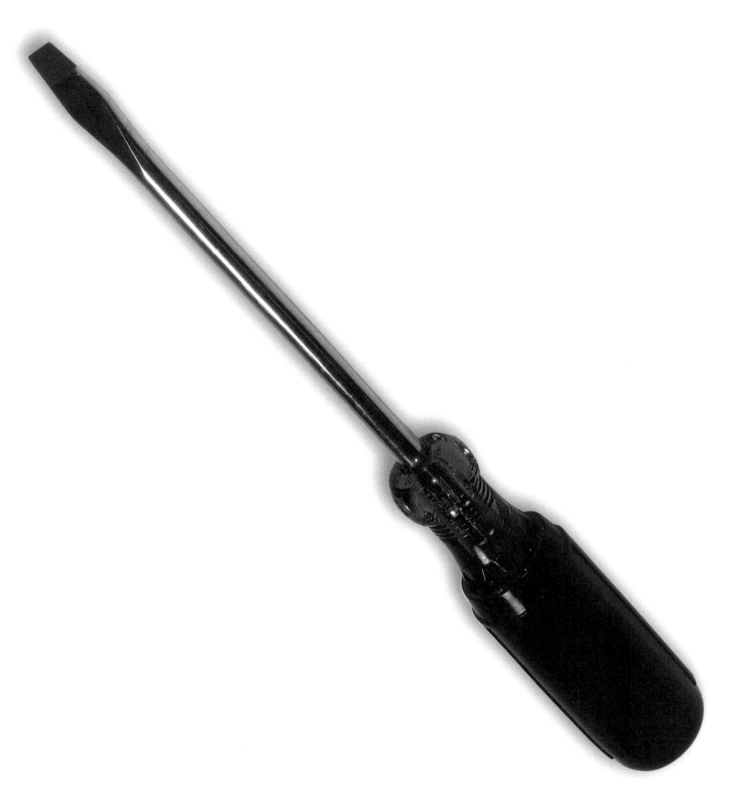

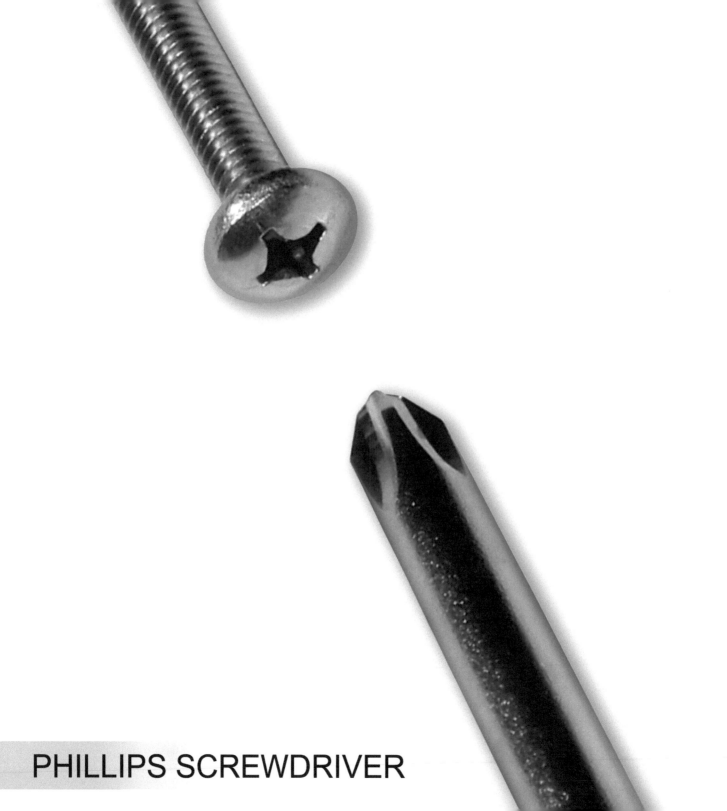

PHILLIPS SCREWDRIVER

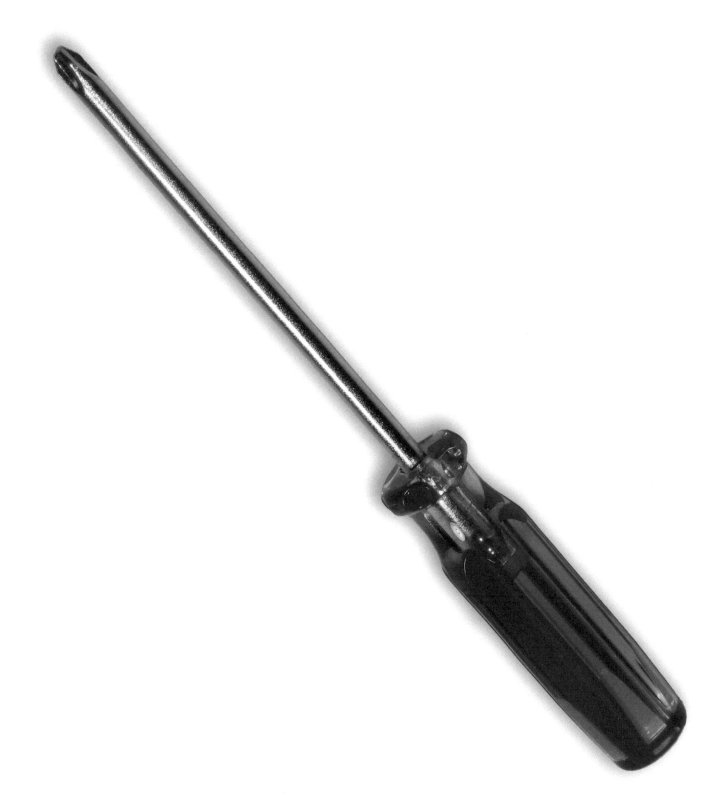

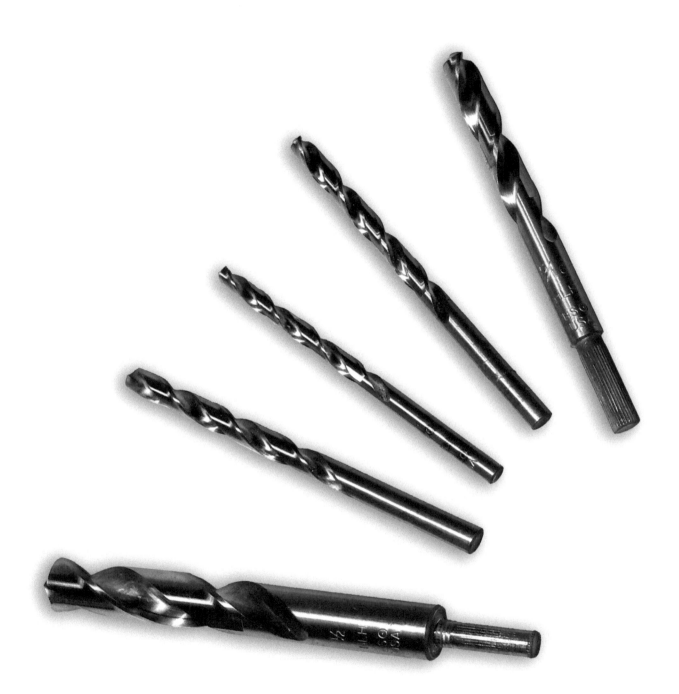

DRILL

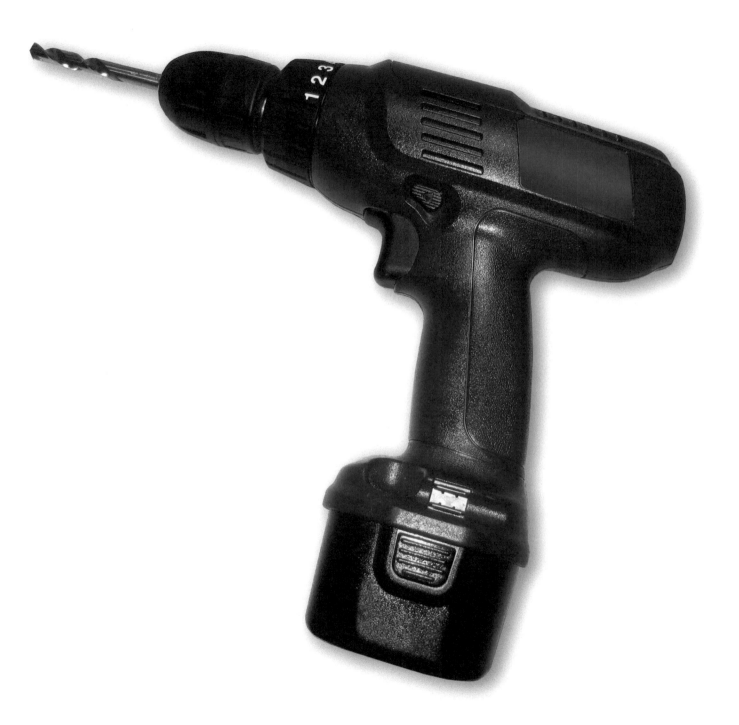

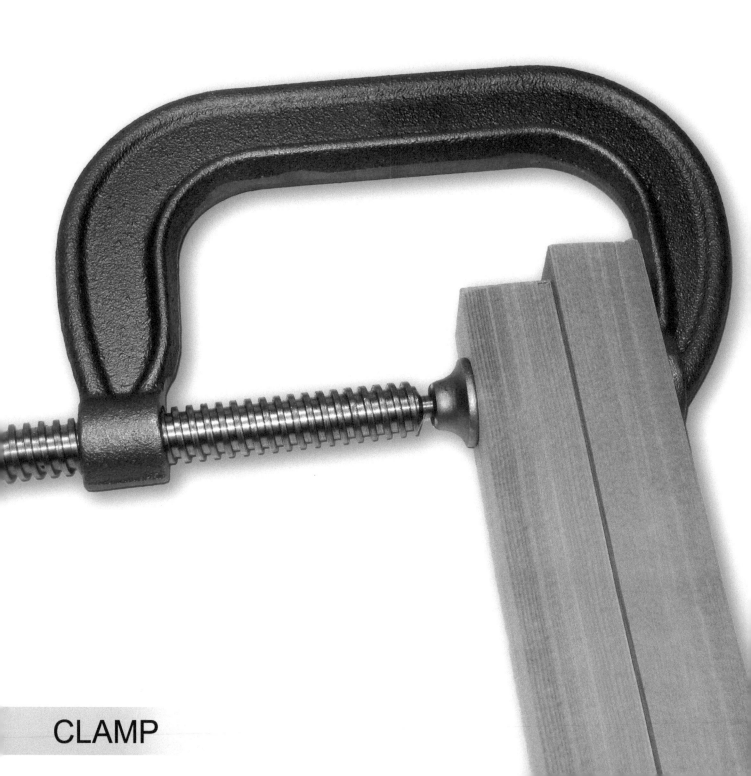

CLAMP

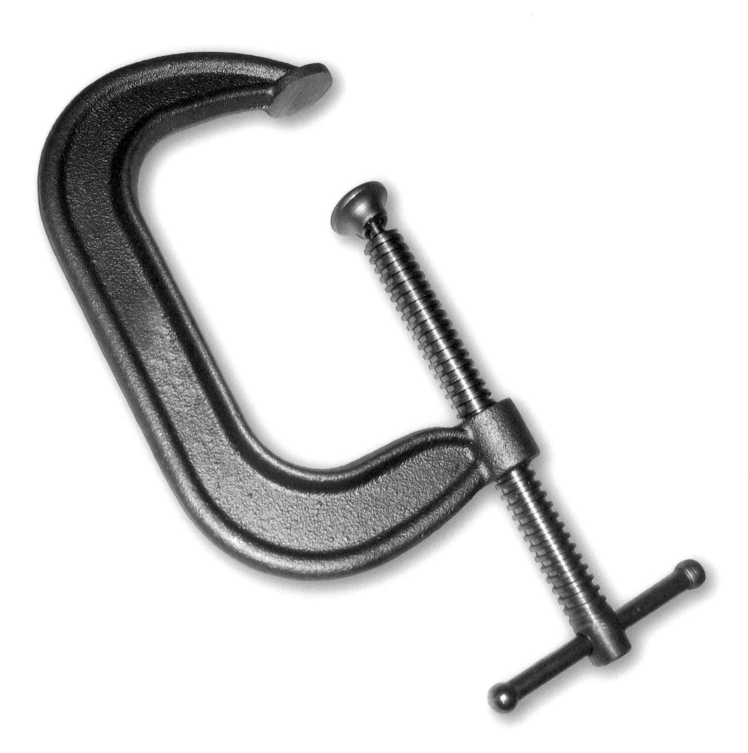

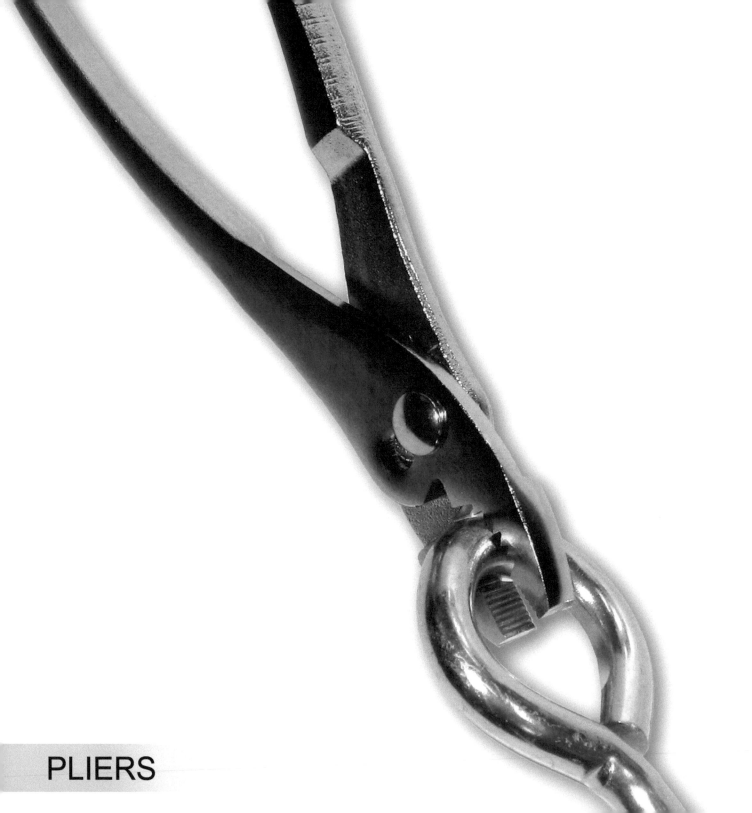

PLIERS

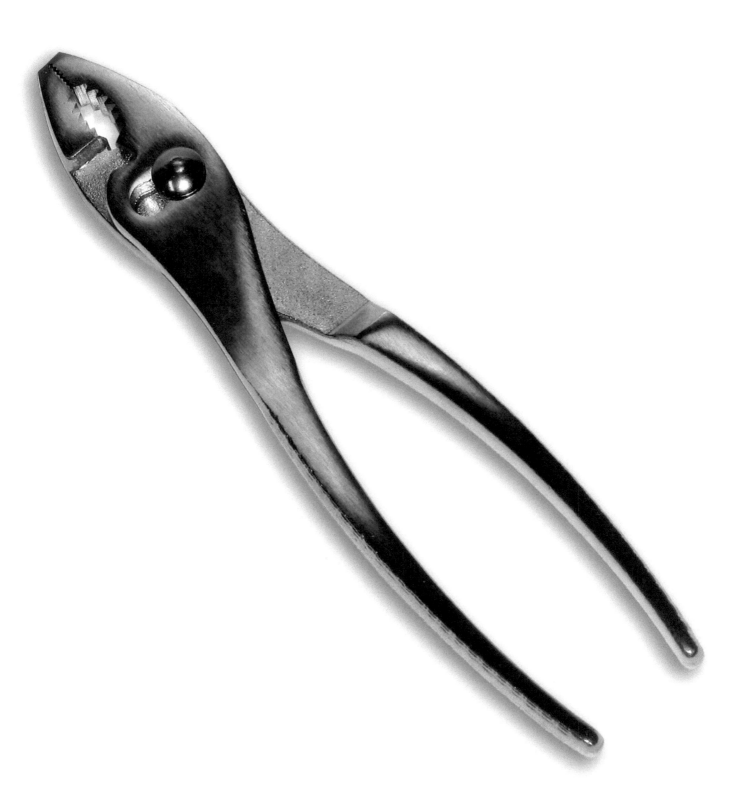

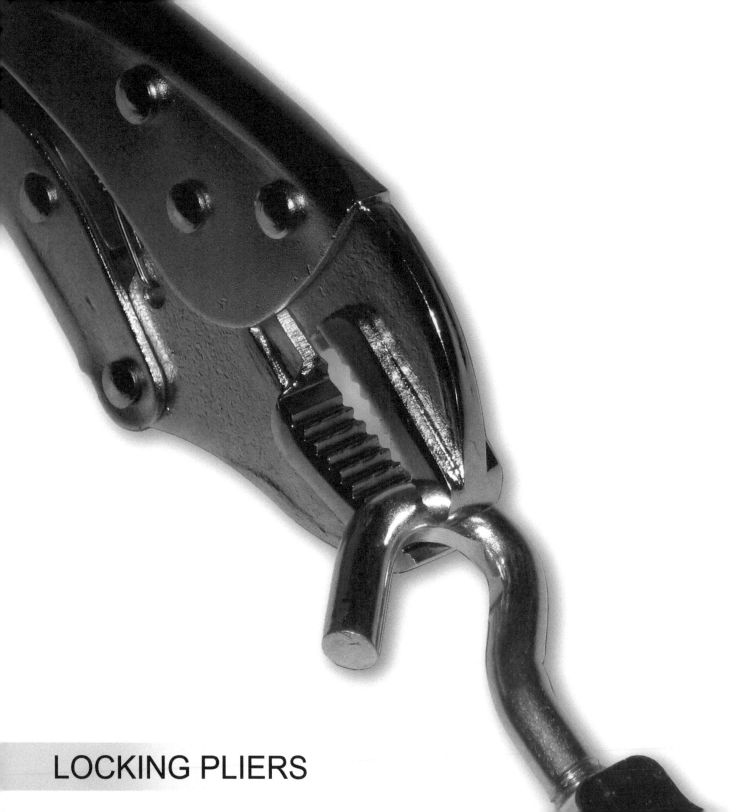

LOCKING PLIERS

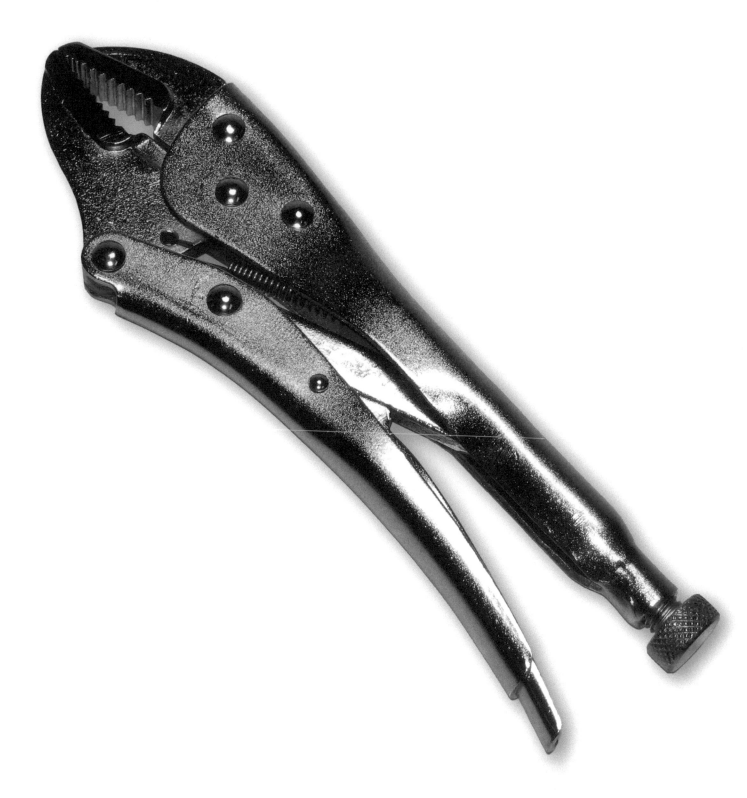

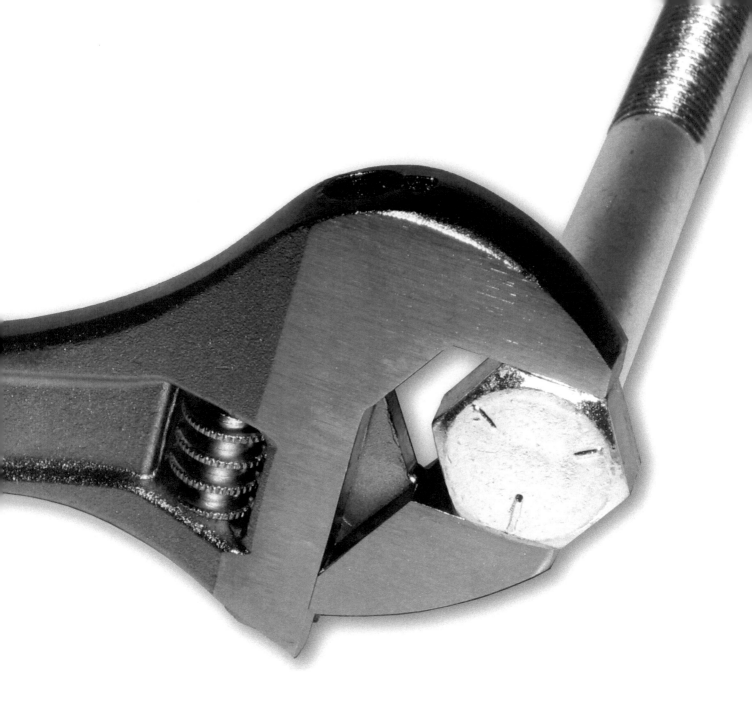

ADJUSTABLE WRENCH

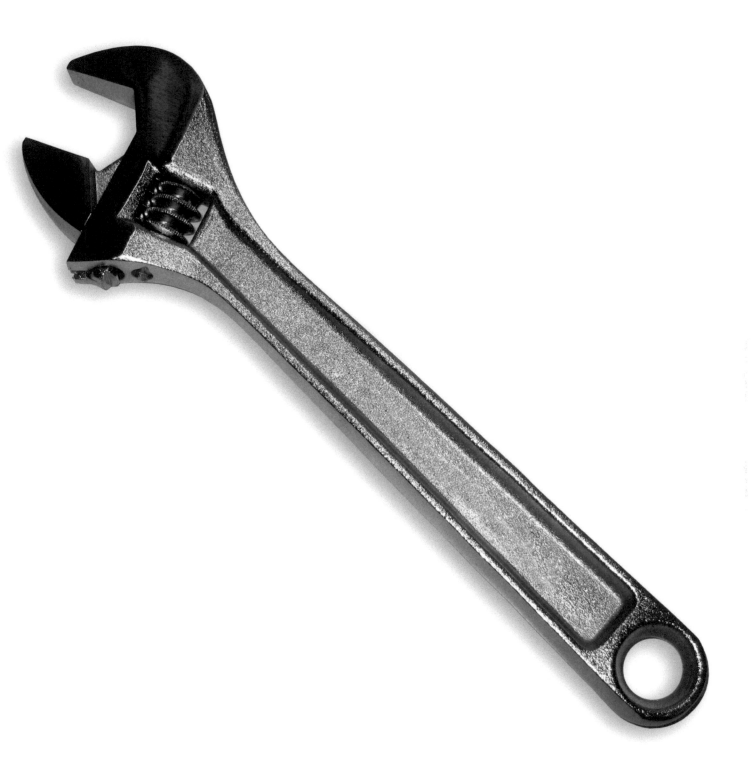

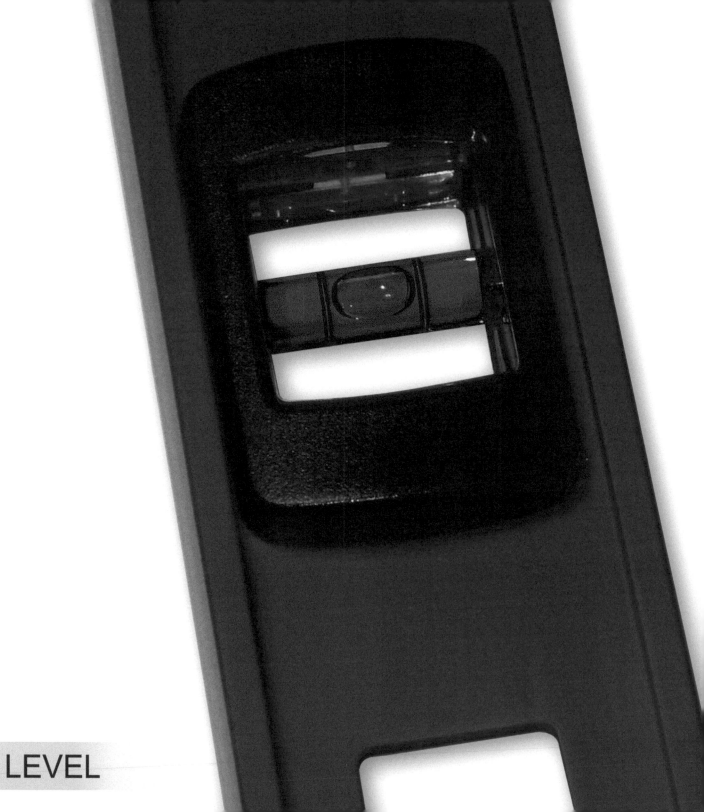

LEVEL

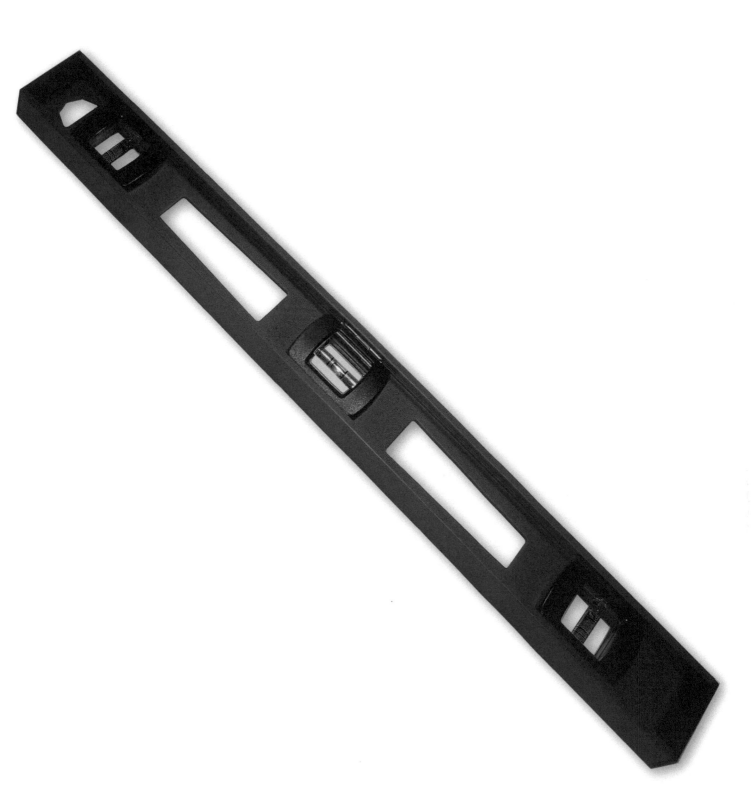

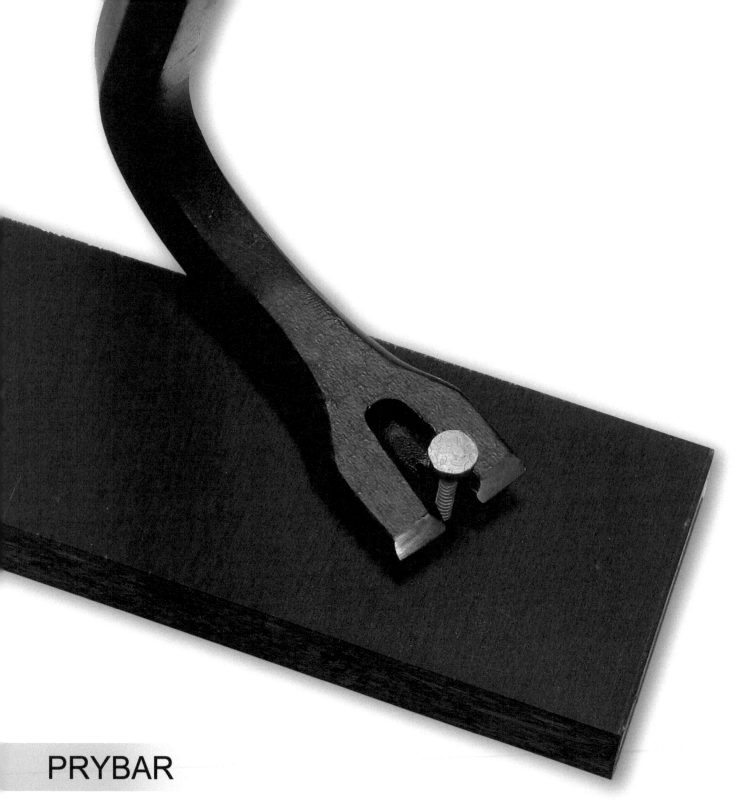

PRYBAR

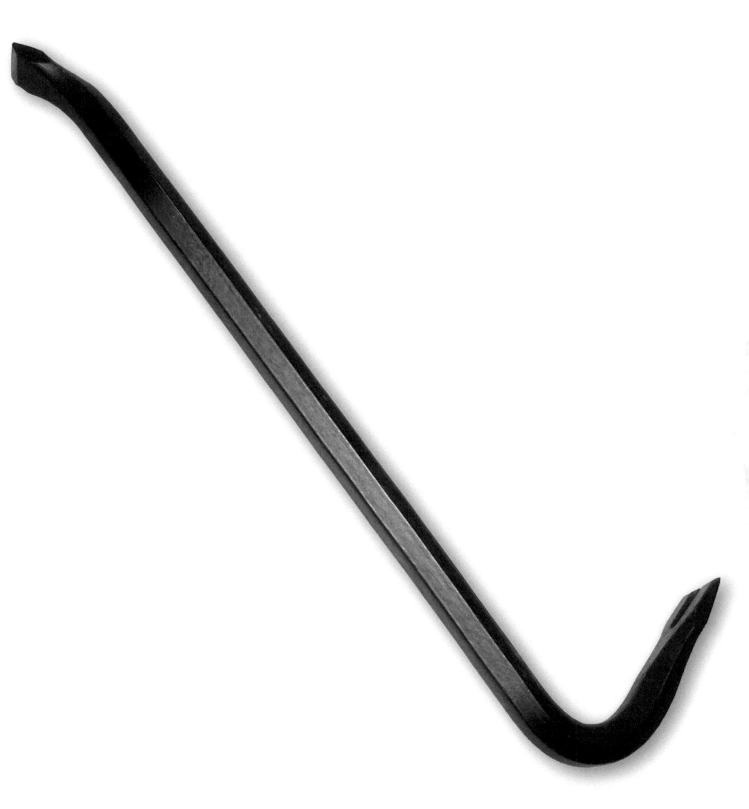

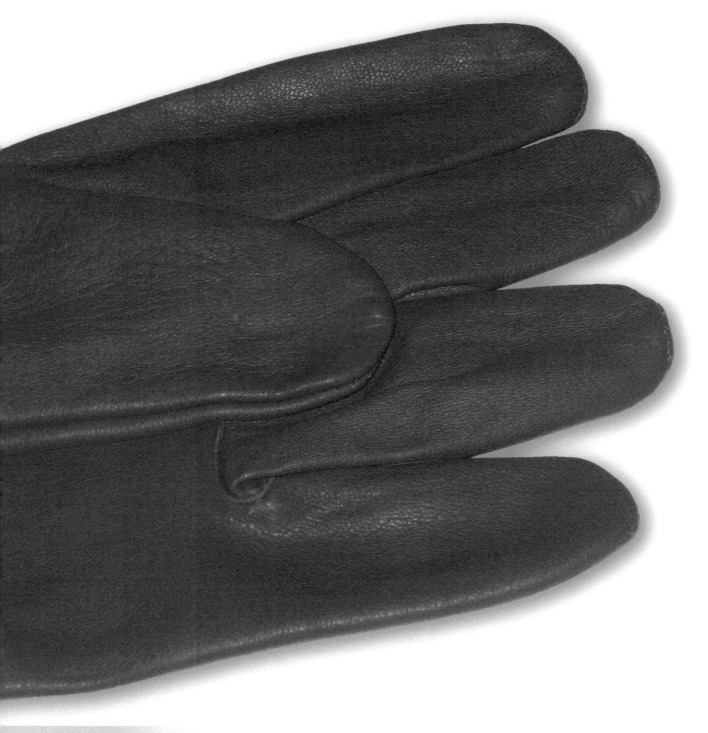

WORK GLOVES

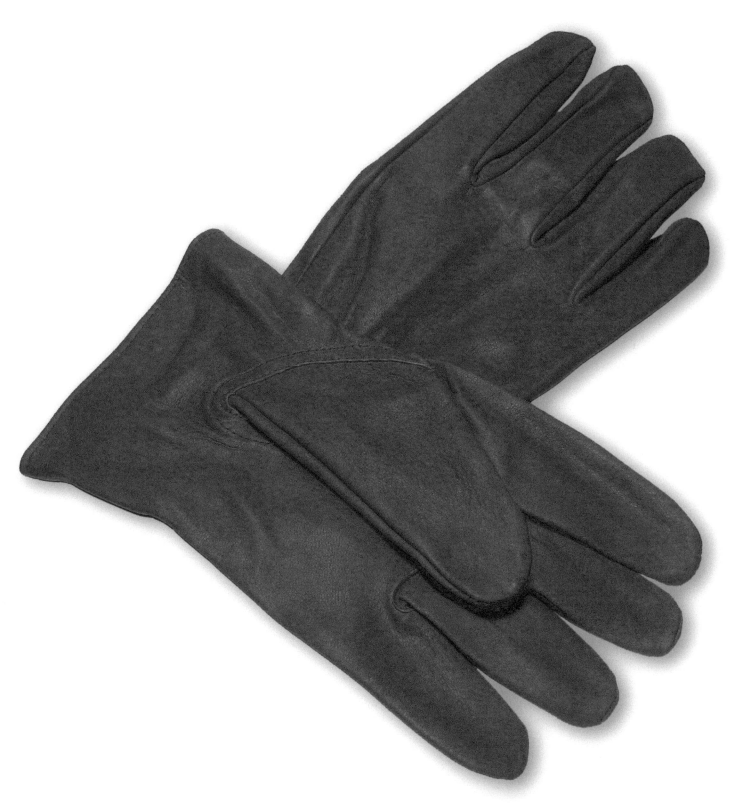

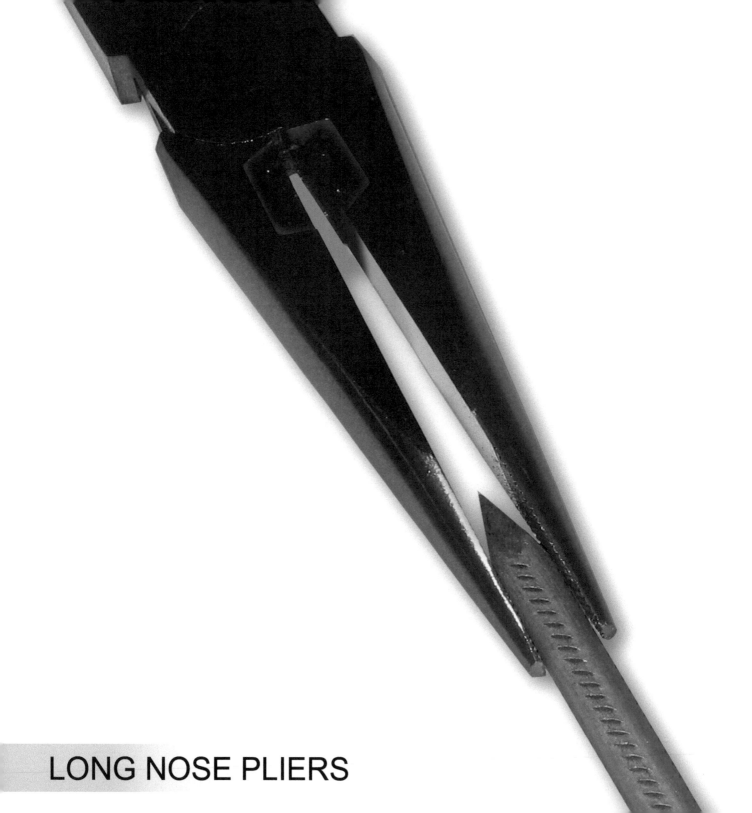

LONG NOSE PLIERS

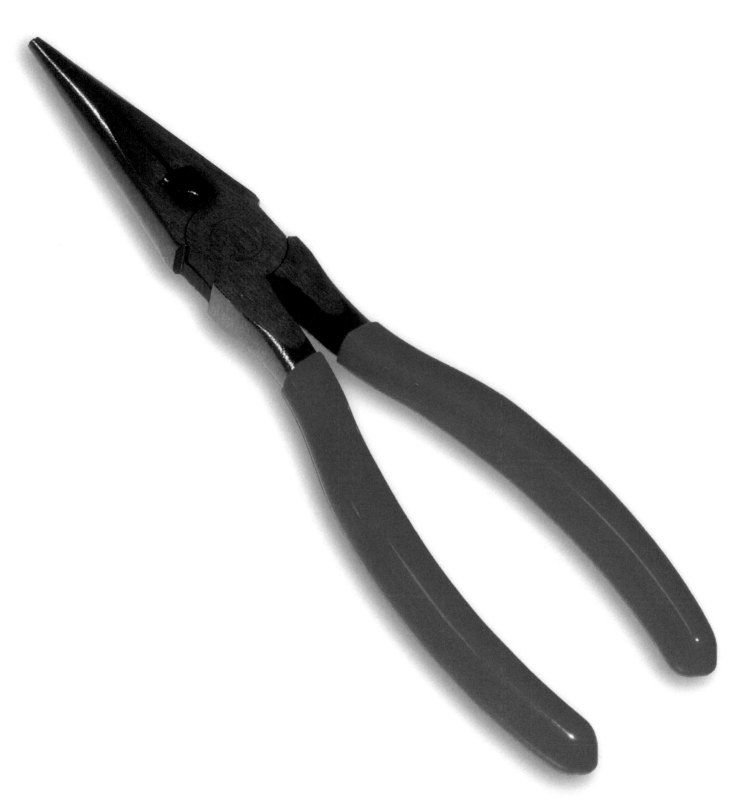

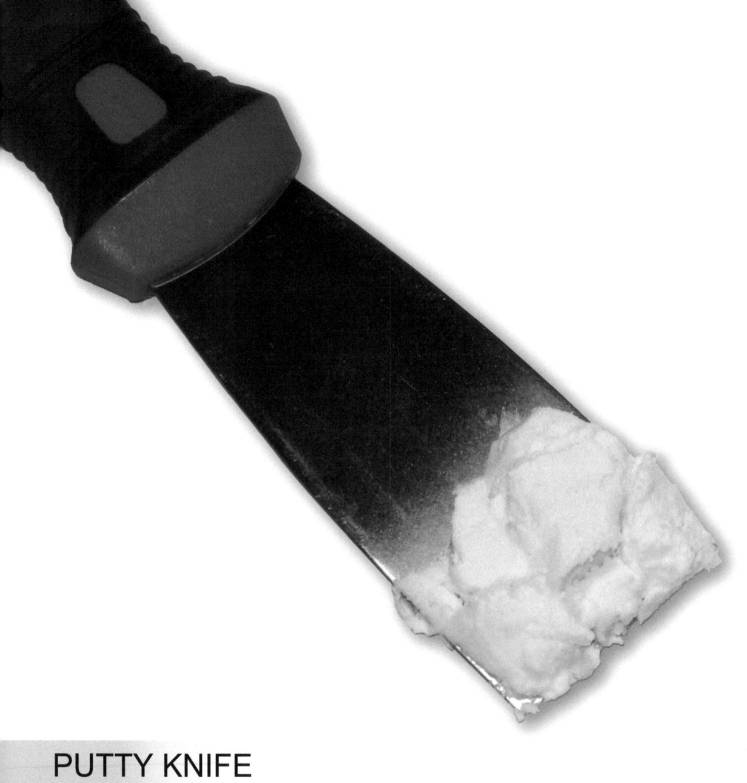

PUTTY KNIFE

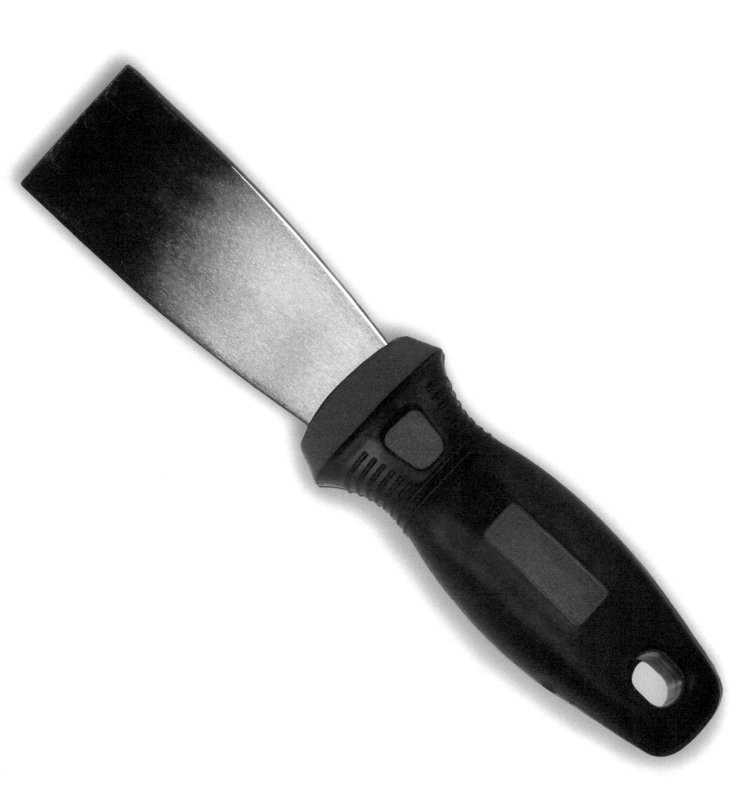

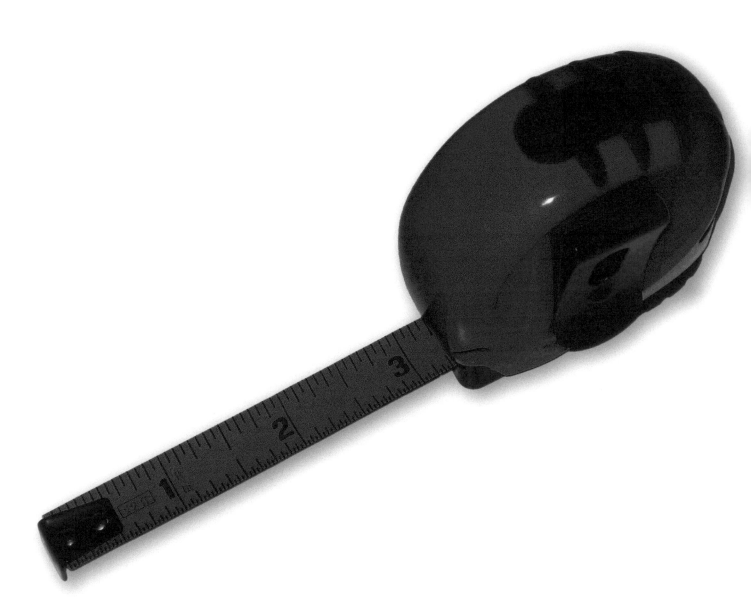

TAPE MEASURE

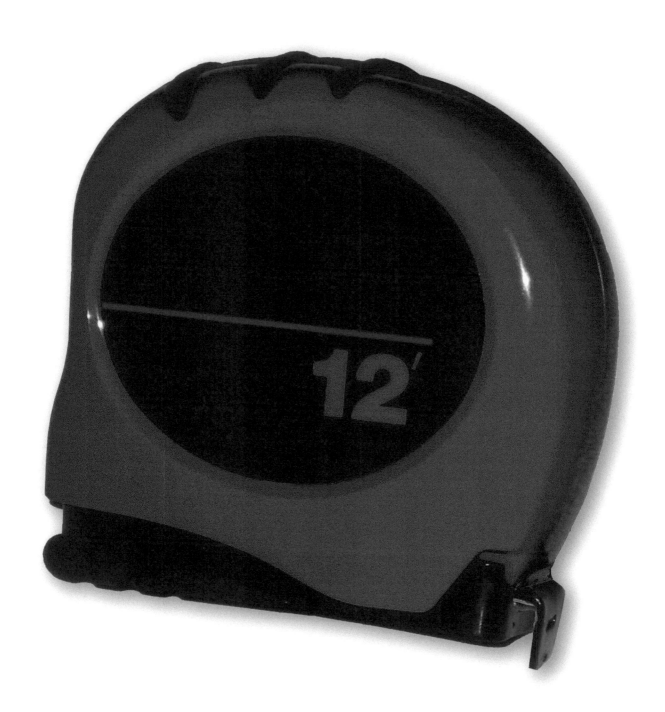

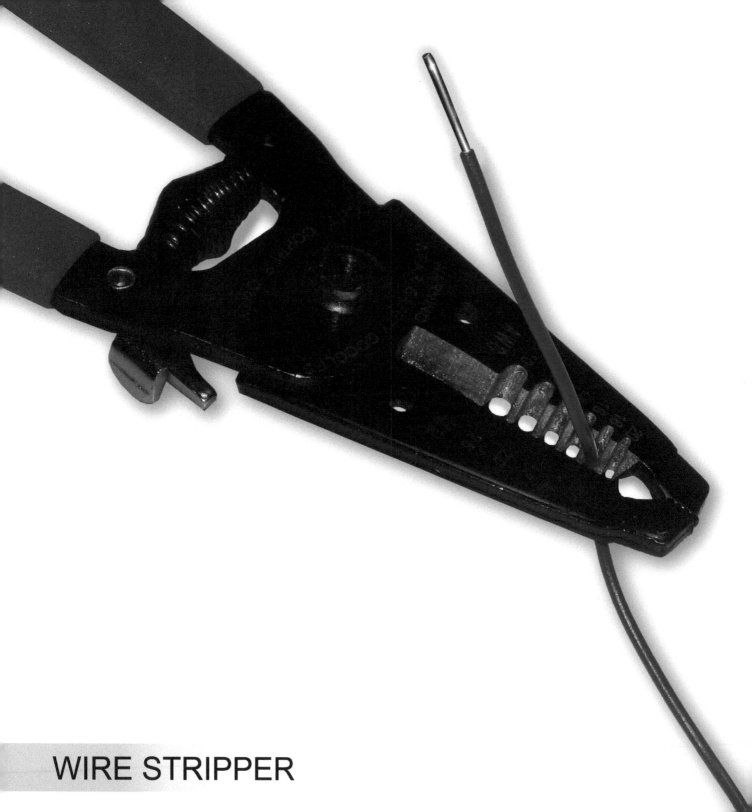

WIRE STRIPPER

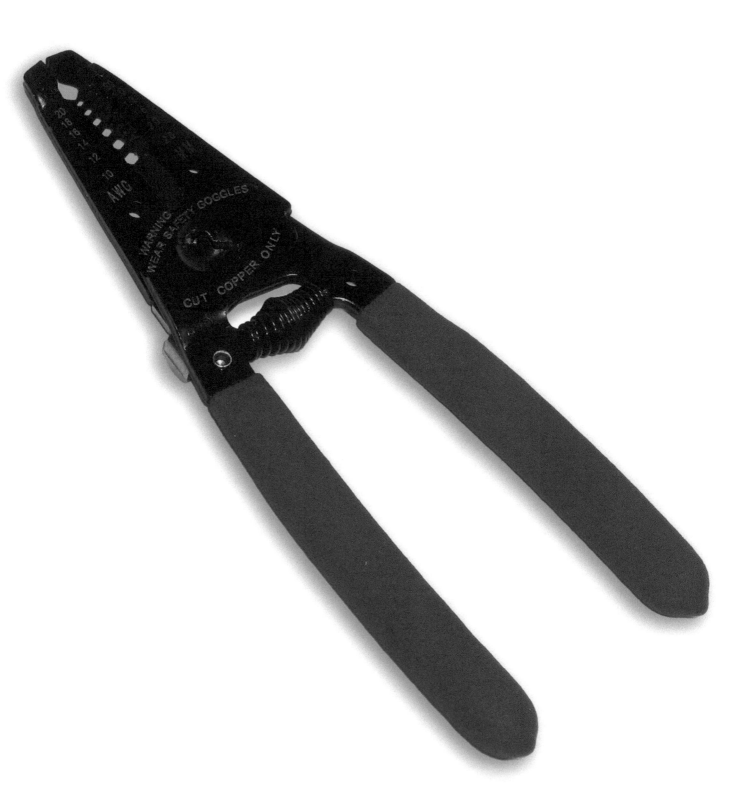

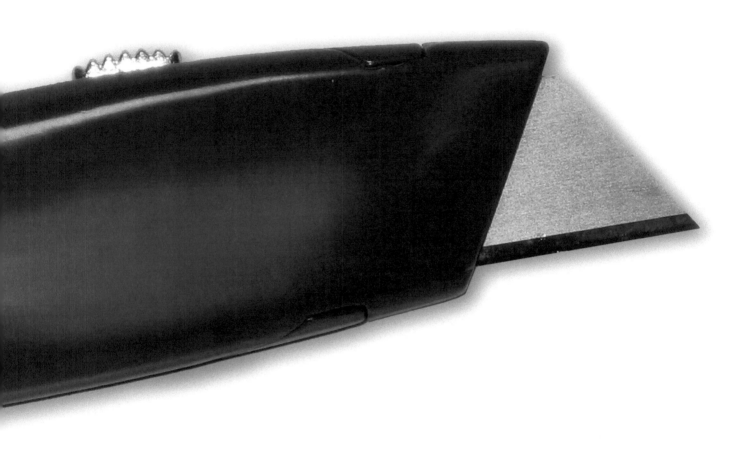

RAZOR CUTTER

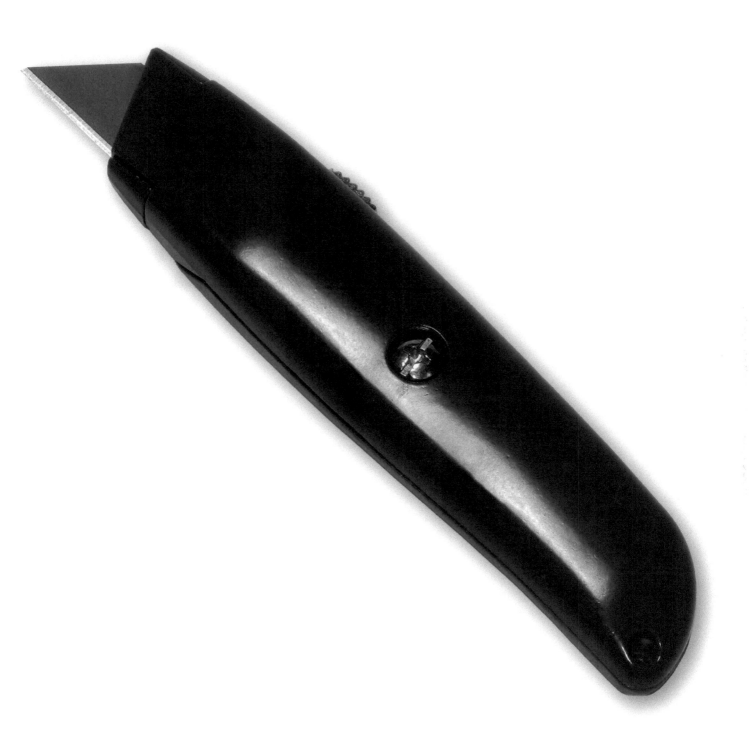

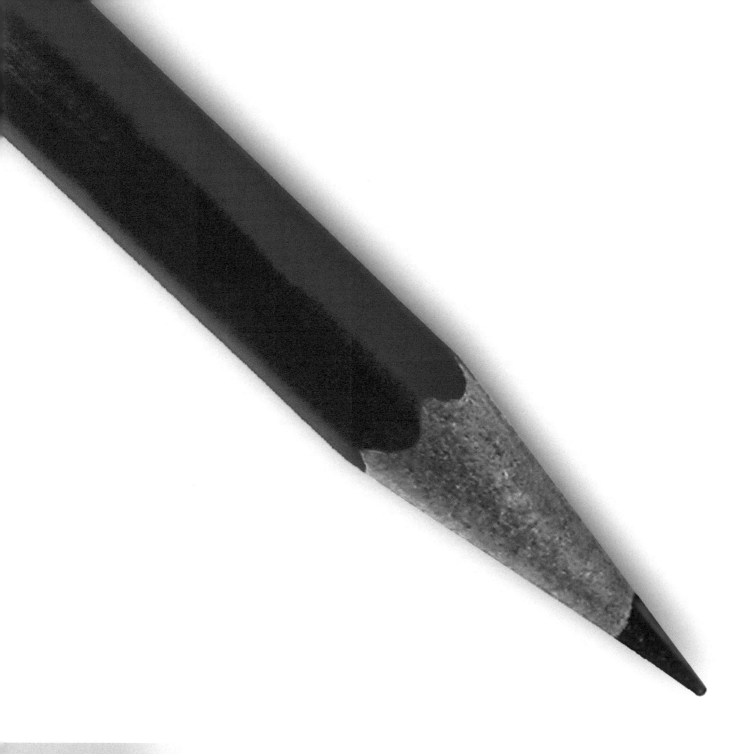

PENCIL

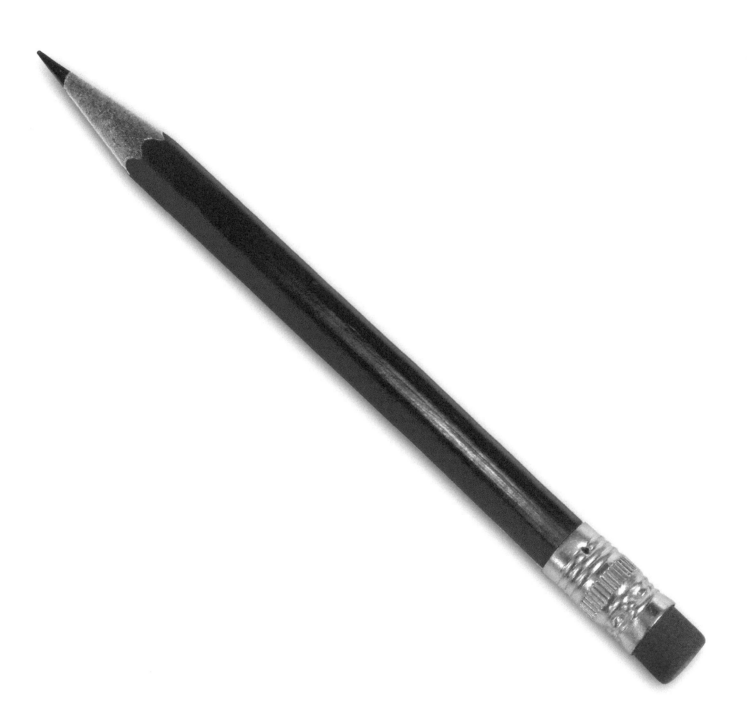

Personalize with other favorite HAND TOOLS

Personalize with other favorite HAND TOOLS

About the Author, Dan Koffman

Dan Koffman is a creative communicator. He believes that art is communication and that the artist has the privilege of choosing what is to be communicated.

Throughout his more than 45 year career, he has communicated as a graphic, commercial and fine artist, designer and marketer of consumer products, community activist and, now, as creator of *Simple Pleasures for Special Seniors*©.

Born in 1950 in Los Angeles, California, Koffman focused first on industrial design and architecture, winning a Gold Medal for his building designs at the California State Fair in 1966 and serving as a draftsman on the Mariner Mars Project – all before completing high school.

From 1970 to 1990 he applied his bold and colorful artistic style to over 1000 internationally marketed consumer products for his company, Bibi Products, Incorporated.

In 1990 he established Bottomline Communications, an international advertising agency in Monterey, California, working with corporations (including Honeywell, Diners Club, Libbey Glass, Toshiba and financial institutions) worldwide, injecting an unexpected and often humorous twist into otherwise traditional marketing, merchandising and advertising campaigns.

"I have always called my work 'Art with a Smile!'" says Koffman. In the mid-1990s he opened Koffman Gallery where he created 'art that celebrates people's passions'.

Giving back to the world has always been an integral part of Koffman's life. To that end, he designed the Flag of Peace and Freedom, painted for peace with an African elephant and launched the Golden Rule Activist project.

The *Simple Pleasures for Special Seniors*© book series, Koffman believes, is art as communication at its most powerful – using artistic talent to make a positive difference in people's lives.

"The experience of witnessing the progression of my dad's dementia and the toll it extracted on my mom, the primary caregiver, and my family registered deeply in my heart and mind," Koffman says. "I wanted to do something that would have a positive effect on everyone involved. *Simple Pleasures for Special Seniors*© is the realization of that goal."

Dan, his wife Sandy, her mother and their two wonderful dogs live on an island in the Pacific Northwest, surrounded by his studio, art gallery and their gardens.

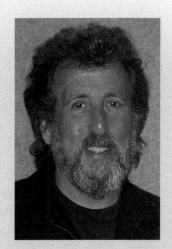

You can learn more about Dan Koffman by visiting his websites:

www.SimplePleasuresforSpecialSeniors.com
Details on upcoming titles.
Hardcover versions of current titles are available directly from the website.

www.artwithasmile.com
Koffman's art that celebrates people's passions.

www.peaceflag.org
Details on the Flag of Peace and Freedom.

www.themanandtheelephant.com
The story of his artistic collaborations with Lisa, the African elephant and their goal of focusing attention on man's relationship and responsibility to animals and to our planet.

www.goldenruleactivist.com
The story of his project to draw attention to the universal message of the Golden Rule.

CPSIA information can be obtained
at www.ICGtesting.com
Printed in the USA
LVHW07n0429170418
573759LV00004B/19/P